# Leptin Resistance:

## Achieve Permanent Weight Loss and Great Health By Understanding Leptin Resistance and the Leptin Hormone

(Leptin Resistance Diet 1)

By Hanna M. Krem

# STOP: READ THIS FIRST

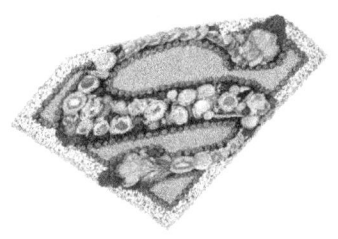

SUPER FRUITS *and* VEGGIES

20 Superfoods That Will Transform Your Health

Hanna M. Krem

Just to say thank you for downloading my book, I would like to give you my 20 Super Fruits And Veggies Report 100% FREE!

DOWNLOAD NOW

(or go to http://www.strengthrecipe.com/free)

**Hanna Krem is a world-class chef and health expert that has setup meal plans and diets for hundreds of thousands of people across the world. As a bonus for purchasing her book, she has added a bonus of the world's BEST super fruits and vegetables that you must eat to gain OPTIMAL health.**

# Table of Content

Error! Not a valid heading level range.

# Chapter 1: What is Leptin?

In terms of clinical health and nutrition, a number of factors, beyond a low calorie diet and exercise, come into play. One of the most discussed principles of health among clinical nutritionists today revolves around the leptin hormone. While many people have never heard of leptin, this hormone is one of the most powerful forces in the body and influences virtually every act that takes place within the system. Those who want to achieve permanent weight loss and great overall health must understand how the leptin hormone works as well as the condition known as leptin resistance that prevents many from losing weight and staying fit.

Leptin is heavily involved with weight management and the body's ability to control its hunger. This means if there is an issue regarding leptin levels in the body it can seem virtually impossible for any person to reach their health and weight loss goals. Studies have shown that when there is an absence of leptin in the body, or when the body has developed leptin resistance, that it can lead to weight gain and uncontrolled eating. Leptin is a very complex hormone, and it can trace back to virtually any function within the body that uses energy. However, for those looking to lose weight and keep that weight off, understanding how this hormone works and how it impacts the body is an essential component of their success.

# Leptin 101: Understanding the Hormone

While there are leptin supplements on the market, leptin itself is a naturally occurring hormone within the body. Many call leptin the "fat hormone" or the "obesity hormone" while other experts refers to it as the "starvation hormone." No matter what the nickname may be, this protein, which is made in the fat cells of the body, has a major impact on weight and appetite.

At a basic level, leptin is a hormone that sends signals to the cells and helps the body to regulate appetite, manage body weight and control food intake. Leptin is also in control of helping the brain regulate how much energy the body has, needs and uses. Leptin can increase activity in the sympathetic nervous system. This is the area of the body that stimulates fatty tissues to burn off energy and extra stored fat within the body.

Leptin also plays an important role in inhibiting the appetite in the hypothalamus. It can do this by sending messages to the receptors in the appetite portion of the brain. This means the hormone can actually regulate and impact the cells in the brain that tell a person how much they need to eat.

As a result, if a person has a proper balance of leptin in the body, or properly functioning leptin hormones, they can easily control their cravings and food intake and effectively burn off extra energy, or calories. If leptin is not functioning properly, a person can have issues controlling how much they eat and how many calories they are able to burn off, even when they are trying to lose weight. This is precisely why those struggling to maintain a healthy weight need to be well versed on the basics of leptin and leptin resistance.

# How Leptin Operates in the Body

Researchers can go into great detail regarding the way leptin travels throughout the body and impacts virtually every system. However, for the average individual, understanding the basic way in which leptin works, travels and influences cells in regards to weight loss and appetite control, is sufficient in helping them understand and eventually overcome a leptin-related issue.

Leptin is actually made within the body's white adipose tissue, or where the body stores fat. What many do not realize is that the stored fat in the body is more than just a place to hold extra calories, it is a thriving metabolic organ, similar to the adrenal or thyroid glands. This means issues with leptin production from the adipose tissues can develop, just as adrenal or thyroid issues can develop and impact the way the body releases these hormones. After leptin is released, it travels through the blood and to the brain. When it does, the hormone delivers a message to the brain regarding how much fuel, or energy the body has to burn.

The easiest way to think about this message is to view it is as the gas gauge for the body. The leptin's message tells the body how much gas it has, and whether it can keep running or needs to stop and fill up the tank. If the leptin gas gauge message is telling the brain that the body is low on fuel, the brain sends a message to eat more or to "fuel up." When a person has eaten enough food, or given the body enough energy, the leptin gauge rises and tells the brain that the energy levels, or tank, are full.

Once the brain receives a signal from the leptin, indicating the energy levels are full, it then gives permission for the metabolism to start running faster. When the brain receives a signal that leptin levels or low, then it tells the metabolism to slow down or to hibernate, so the body doesn't waste away from malnutrition. It doesn't matter if the person has eaten or if there is food available, the brain will assume that there is a famine and that the metabolism needs to shut down for preservation.

With this in mind, it is easy to see why leptin is considered to be such as powerful hormone. Leptin is in control of the rate in which the human body makes energy, which is essential to virtually every thing the body does, including maintaining a healthy weight. Leptin is also entirely in control of what the brain tells the body in terms of how hungry a person is or how much food they need to be eating.

Leptin is powerful, and it is an important component to a successfully functioning body. This is also why a leptin issue can so easily impact the body's ability to function and cause issues that go far beyond packing on a few extra pounds. Leptin also plays a role in how the immune system functions, regulating the basic functions of the brain, the thyroid, adrenal functions, reproductive capabilities and stress. With so much riding on properly functioning leptin hormones, it is essential that every person understands how leptin works, know how to spot leptin issues and learns what happens when this hormone stops functioning in the way it is intended to.

# When Leptin Doesn't Work

Many people will never have an issue with leptin. It is a powerful and very complex hormone that operates in the even more complex system of the human body. Many times, the body is able to compensate for small issues and "fix itself" when something such as leptin hormone regulation is off. However, there are other times when, for a number of reasons, leptin can stop working in the way it is supposed to entirely.

One of the most common and basic problems related to leptin occurs when the leptin "gas gauge" is broken or not working, as it is intended to. This is similar to a malfunctioning or "stuck" gas gauge that is stuck on the "E" line, even when the actual tank is full. This issue typically has nothing to do with the amount of leptin being released in the body, but instead how that leptin is reading its fuel gauge. This unfortunately is very common in overweight individuals, as their leptin gauge is telling their subconscious drive to eat more food than they need in order to feel satisfied and to fuel the body.

While animal studies have shown that many obese mice have low levels of leptin and benefit tremendously from extra leptin in the system, unfortunately many obese individuals actually have an excess level of leptin in their system. This means while there are some leptin capsules and injections available on the market, these will not help any leptin related problems. In many situations, the issue typically is not regarding the amount of leptin but that the leptin in the body is not functioning, as it should.

# Chapter 2: Leptin Resistance

When an individual has a normal or high amount of leptin circulating in their bloodstream, but are struggling with obesity, chances are they have what is known as leptin resistance. The term "leptin resistance" actually doesn't indicate an issue with the amount of leptin in the body; it simply means that the body is not responding to the hormone in the way it is designed to. While there is some individuals whose bodies may not be producing enough leptin, in most situations, struggles with weight loss are actually dealing with this leptin resistance. While this condition is very common and often very frustrating as it can make it seem impossible to lose weight, there are ways to overcome leptin resistance.

The key to doing this is to know the signs and symptoms of this issue, knowing why leptin resistance happens and implementing a new diet that helps individuals overcome their leptin related issues.

# What it Means to Have Leptin Resistance

When an individual is labeled as leptin resistant, it basically means even though the leptin in their system is sending a message to the brain, the brain is essentially ignoring what the leptin is saying. Many equate resistant to this type of hormone as being similar to "The Boy Who Cried Wolf." The leptin is crying so much, that the brain starts to ignore the cries, much like people started to ignore the boy in the fable.

When the body gains weight and fat, the adipose tissues, where this fat is stored, starts to produce more and more leptin. However, it can reach a point where there is so much leptin being produced that the messages sent from the leptin can get ignored, which is similar to the way the body responds to having too much insulin. In the case of leptin, when this happens, the body thinks that it is starving since its not getting any signals from the hormone stating that its "fuel gauge" is full. Essentially, the brain is receiving the opposite message it is supposed to, and instead of the metabolism springing into action to start burning off extra fuel, the body thinks that it is starving. The metabolism then shuts down, goes into hibernation mode and starts preserving energy to ward of famine.

This is why so many people who are leptin resistant not only struggle with obesity but they struggle to ever overcome this obesity. The body becomes confused regarding how much food it needs to survive and when it needs to be burning off the extra fuel in its system and becomes stuck in a state of feeling hungry yet still feeling the need to preserve fat and energy.

For the many people struggling with leptin resistance, one of the biggest questions they have is "how does leptin resistance happen?" Unfortunately, there is not a definitive cause of leptin resistance, but experts have two primary hypotheses regarding how this lack of communication happens. One hypothesis is that the leptin in the blood is, for some reason, unable to reach the proper targets, or place in the brain that controls the appetite. Another guess that experts have is that the receptors in the body that leptin proteins are supposed to bind to stop functioning in the right way, meaning they are unable to tell the cells how to respond to the presence of the hormone properly. No matter how this miscommunication happens, what is most important is the why this issue starts to occur.

# Factors That Contribute to Leptin Resistance

No matter what the cause is for these hormones to stop functioning properly, there are several known factors that tend to contribute to leptin resistance issues. As with most other hormone issues, experts typically cannot pinpoint a single factor that causes leptin resistance. Many believe that the body develops leptin resistance much like it develops insulin resistance, meaning that the body becomes resistant to the hormone by continuous high exposure to the hormone.

While some individuals may unknowingly cause their body to produce too much leptin and therefore develop a leptin resistance, other healthy individuals may also naturally start to become resistant to leptin for unknown reasons. However, studies on the topic have shown there are several factors that may contribute to the body's tendency to ignore leptin signals.

Stress and Lifestyle Issues

Stress and lifestyle choices can contribute to problems with leptin resistance. Research shows that individuals who have high stress levels are more likely to have hormonal imbalances. Individuals who do not get enough sleep also may be at a higher risk of developing leptin issues. People with high insulin levels have also been shown to be more likely to have leptin resistance, as these two hormones tend to go hand-in-hand.

Pre-existing Issues

Several pre-existing issues within the body can cause leptin resistance. Inflammation in the hypothalamus can cause leptin resistance. Those who begin with high levels of leptin in their body are also more likely to develop leptin resistance. People with an elevated level of free fatty acids in the blood; typically also have more fat metabolites in their brain, which can impact leptin signals. These are all factors that can occur in any individual, but they are factors that are increased in obese individuals.

Dietary Choices

A poor diet can contribute to issues with leptin communicating with the brain in the way that it is supposed to. Studies show that consuming an excessive amount of simple carbs, overeating, and grain and lectin consumption can all contribute to leptin resistance issues. Also high amounts of fructose consumption, particularly with High Fructose Corn Syrup can cause the body to stop responding to leptin appropriately. Diets high in sugars such as this get metabolized in the body's fat cells; the same cells that release leptin. Maintaining a diet such as this can cause the fat cells to produce too much leptin and cause the body to start becoming resistant to the hormone.

Exercise Contributions

A healthy lifestyle that includes a balanced diet and plenty of exercise is a great way to keep the body functioning in the way it should, and many times it can prevent issues regarding leptin resistance from developing. However, some studies indicate that exercising too much can actually lead to issues with leptin resistance, especially if an individual is exercising excessively when their hormones are already damaged. This contributing factor to leptin resistance can be nearly impossible to control or regulate, but this extra stress on the hormones can in-fact prevent leptin from functioning as it should.

While none of these contributing factors will necessarily cause leptin problems, they can all increase an individual's chance of developing this type of hormonal de-sensitivity. Individuals who live a life with several of these contributing factors, and also struggle with appetite control and weight loss likely already have a case of leptin-resistance.

# Chapter 3: Diagnosing Leptin Resistance

The key to overcoming leptin resistance is to first determine whether or not a leptin problem is really at the core of these health issues. Many times the signs of this imbalance are the same as other common ailments, which makes getting an actual leptin resistance diagnosis isn't always easy. The good news is, once someone knows they are leptin resistant, they can easily start implementing diet and lifestyle changes that can reestablish their sensitivity to this hormone.

Many experts believe that leptin resistance may be the one primary biological abnormality in obese individuals. This is why obese people are the most susceptible to leptin resistance issues. This happens because of the relatively simple cycle of leptin development. Obese individuals have a great deal of body fat stored within their fat cells. These fat cells produce leptin in proportion to their size, meaning the more fat the more leptin. This is why obese individuals tend to have extremely high levels of leptin in their body. Based on the way the leptin hormone is supposed to operate, these individuals should not be over eating. The brain should know the body has plenty of energy in its tank and that it doesn't need any more fuel. However with leptin resistance, this signal stops working and the message gets lost.

When this happens, the body becomes resistant to leptin much like it becomes resistant to insulin when there's too much floating around. When the brain stops receiving leptin signals, it thinks the body is starved, even if there is enough energy available, or stored within the body. This is why the brain thinks obese individuals need to eat and why the metabolism needs to slow down to conserve energy. This is precisely why overweight individuals are the most susceptible for having leptin resistance and why they have so much of an issue breaking the cycle.

# Signs and Symptoms of Leptin Resistance

There are a number of ways in which leptin resistance issues present themselves in the body. This can make noticing some of the signs and symptoms of this issue difficult for individuals to spot. Many people may attribute these signs as issues simply related to being overweight. However, those who do struggle with weight and who are serious about overcoming their battle with weight loss will want to pay close attention to the following signs and symptoms. Spotting a potential issue with leptin resistance can help any person overcome this problem and get on a path that will help their body get back to functioning in the healthy manner it is supposed to. These are some of the most common symptoms of leptin resistance:

Irritability and mood swings
High weight and excess fat on the body
Carbohydrate cravings, particularly at night
Large appetite and the tendency to over eat
Insomnia and fatigue

High cholesterol, blood sugar or
triglycerides
Allergies and food sensitivities
Persistent adult acne

Many times individuals who are leptin resistant
also have other conditions including thyroid
issues and a condition known as fatty liver.
Women with this hormonal problem are also
more likely to have ovarian cysts and
endometriosis.

# How to Diagnose Someone as Leptin Resistant

Diagnosing leptin resistance is a difficult task, as a person can have low, normal or high levels of leptin in their blood stream, yet still be either leptin resistant or have completely normal leptin function. With this in mind, there are a few ways to determine if an individual has a leptin resistance issue. First, it is essential to remember that a person can be leptin resistant whether they are overweight, average or underweight. However, if an individual is overweight by more than 30 pounds, it's almost a guarantee that they are leptin resistant in some way. Individuals, who are excessively underweight, typically by 20 pounds or more, are often also leptin resistant.

This is often one of the easiest ways to diagnose this type of hormonal resistance, but for others who desire a more accurate reading, or who are not sure based on their weight, there is a blood test. A simple blood test is typically around 90% accurate. There are a handful of blood tests available to help determine leptin resistance, but two of the most common are HS CRP, which looks for highly sensitive C-Reactive proteins, or the T3 blood test. There is another salivary cortisol test that is performed every 15 minutes for one whole hour after eating. With a leptin resistance diagnosis, it can be easier to determine the proper course of action to start restoring leptin sensitivity.

# Common Side Effects of Being Leptin Resistant

When an individual is dealing with a serious issue with leptin resistance, they may notice additional side effects in addition to some of the common signs and symptoms they may have noticed in the past. One of the biggest side effects of a prolonged issue with leptin sensitivity is that the metabolism starts to slow down. Leptin also impacts the thyroid and when the leptin is not transmitting messages properly, the thyroid often stops releasing the hormones that speed up the metabolism. This leaves many people with a lower amount of energy and the inability to burn off stored fat, even with exercise.

Many individuals with this issue complain that it takes them a very long time to get full, and that they never get the sensation of being full while they are eating. Eventually, many of these people over eat in excess until their stomach is physically unable to hold any more food. They typically do this until they wind up feeling uncomfortably stuffed. Many individuals with this condition also have a heightened reaction to sweets. With leptin problems, the tongue can actually lose some of its sensitivity to sweet foods, meaning items that may once have seemed sweet or even overly sweet, no longer taste the same. Ultimately, it also means it takes more sugar or sweeter foods to satisfy the individual.

# Chapter 4: Overcoming and Treating Leptin Resistance

Unfortunately for those dealing with leptin resistance issues, there is no one magic pill that can restore leptin function. There are however, several steps that individuals can take to help overcome their resistance to leptin and treat this ailment. Restoring leptin sensitivity can take a long time. A leptin resistance typically develops over a period of several years, and when this much long-term damage has been done, it can take a while to reverse it. While the process does take time, it is important to remember that the best approach is a multi-faceted one, and an approach that entails several steps, tactics and lifestyle changes. Just making one small change, typically won't do the trick. Restoring leptin function requires many changes, and necessitates long-term dedication to the cause.

# Lifestyle Changes That Can Improve Leptin Resistance Issues

While there are countless ways to help improve the body's leptin response, one of the first and easiest things anyone with a leptin resistance issue can do is to start making changes to their routine and everyday lifestyle. While dietary changes also need to be made, starting with these changes in routine can help expedite the body's recovery process.

## Getting Sleep

It is very important for an individual struggling with proper leptin response to get enough sleep, but unfortunately it is something that many people do not take seriously enough. Getting to bed early and getting quality, undisturbed sleep, is one of the best things that someone with leptin resistance issues can do. Quality sleep helps the body naturally heal itself, and it helps decrease stress levels. Starting with sleep is a great way for any person to help get these hormones balanced, and operating in the way they were intended to.

Consistent Exercise

Smart exercise is essential to healthy metabolic function and it helps active that genes that promote proper leptin function. The key to smart exercise when rebuilding leptin sensitivity is to focus on consistency. This is far more important than intensity. Walking 30 minutes every day is more beneficial than running six miles once or twice a week. A workout that is too intense will only add extra stress on the body.

Intermitten Fasting

The process of intermitted fasting is one that not only helps people lose weight, but one that can help the body reset and allows it to heal. This is important for giving the body time to heal and recover from the past damage that has caused leptin resistance. While many people will try to fast for a few days as an extreme dieting approach, intermitted fasting is essentially doing a small fast every day to achieve similar metabolic results. The key is to try to leave at least a 12-hour gap between the last meal of one day and the first meal of the next.

# Foods to Avoid When Treating Leptin Resistance

There are certain foods that tend to enhance leptin resistance issues. Avoiding these foods at all costs is one of the best ways to treat leptin resistance. The impact of avoiding these foods does not happen overnight, so it is important to remove these foods and keep them out of the diet as much as possible. This can be hard for any person to do, especially those with serious cravings. The best way to find success in taking these foods from the diet is to start slow and remove these items one by one.

Remove the following items from the diet:
Sugars and fructose, such as high fructose corn syrup
Simple starches
Refined foods
Omega-6s such as vegetable oil and conventional grains
Salted, roasted peanuts
Breads, pastries and cakes

Sweets of any kind besides the occasional dark chocolate
Alcohol

Many of these foods are part of most people's everyday diets, but they only feed leptin resistance issues and continue to make the problem worse. When it comes to removing these items from the diet, many will start to have severe symptoms of withdrawal, especially when removing sweets. This is normal, and it will take the body several days to become less dependent on sugars.

# Dietary Supplements

As with any healthy lifestyle overhaul, many people attempt to add dietary supplements to their leptin diet plan. While many can find the results that they need without extra vitamins and supplements, these all-natural supplements can give a leptin re-sensitizing effort the extra boost that it needs. Even though these supplements are natural, and typically rather healthy, it is important that any person who starts taking these supplements regularly consults a medical professional before getting started. Even naturally occurring supplements can interact with other vitamins or medications. When it comes to choosing the right supplements for a leptin diet plan, these are some of the top options to consider.

Omega-3 Supplements

Omega-3 supplements can increase healthy leptin levels and function, as it helps produce glucose.

Zinc

Take zinc tablets to increase your healthy leptin levels, they act much like Omega-3 supplements and can promote proper message transmissions in these hormones.

Irvingia Gabonesis

Recent studies have found that extract from the African plant; Irvingia gabonesis can actually correct leptin resistance issues. This plant also helps jumpstart the metabolism, promotes weight loss and can counteract issues related to metabolic syndrome.

Fish Oil Supplements

Taking fish oil will keep the body's cell membranes healthy and functioning properly. This allows them to better respond to signals from leptin proteins.

Vitamin C

Vitamin C helps prevent some of the adverse effects of sugar from taking place, which is a serious problem for those dealing with leptin resistant issues. Taking vitamin C daily also helps boost the immune system and restore the body's proper function.

Consider any of these supplements as part of a healthy, balanced diet to see the effects of a pro-leptin restoring effort take place even faster.

# Leptin As An Obesity Treatment

One of the most common questions individuals have regarding leptin resistance treatments is using actual leptin hormones as a method to treat obesity. Shortly after leptin was discovered in the 1990s, many experts began testing this theory. This was also before researchers truly understood that leptin and obesity were linked because of leptin resistance not a leptin deficiency.

With some additional studies into the matter, scientists discovered that most obese individuals actually had an excess of leptin in their body. No matter how much extra leptin in added to the system, the resistance would continue to be an issue. There are a number of leptin supplements sold, particularly online, that may promise to aid in weight loss. However, sine leptin is a protein, the body won't be able to break up or absorb the hormone when it is taken in pill form. With this in mind, even though some will attempt to take leptin supplements, ingesting these hormones will not do anything to counteract issues with weight gain and leptin resistance.

# Chapter 5: The Leptin Diet

Individuals who suffer from leptin issues may feel as though there is no way to break the viscous cycle of leptin resistance. Many experts believe that the influence this hormone has on the body is more powerful than willpower alone. This means there is very little chance that deciding to choose to eat healthy alone will reduce the amount of fat in the body and restore leptin function. However, by embracing a specialized diet, known as the leptin diet, any individual can help reset their bodies in a way that can have leptin functioning normally. In addition to making lifestyle changes and avoiding certain potentially detrimental foods, those suffering from leptin resistance can embrace the leptin diet to restore their sensitivity to this hormone.

One of the most important things to remember about the leptin diet is that it is almost as important to eat at the right time, as it is to eat the right things. The secret to this diet is about getting more, healthy energy from less food. This is not a fad diet, it is a sustainable one, meant for long term results in those who truly suffer from leptin resistance. Over time, this diet can start working and while it may not deliver instant weight loss results, it can help decrease fat storage and promote better leptin sensitivity. The most powerful part of this diet is that it not only works for those who are known to have a leptin resistance issue, but it can be a beneficial long-term diet for anyone looking to achieve and sustain a healthy weight.

# The Basic Rules of the Leptin Diet

Before getting started with the leptin diet, it is essential to know the basic rules of this dietary plan. No matter what specific meals you eat, it is important to always attempt to abide by these rules. A great way to stay on track with these rules is to write them out and keep them in a visual place that serves as a constant reminder.

## 1. Eat a Protein-Filled Protein Breakfast

Most people know the old adage "the first meal of the day is the most important." This saying especially holds true when it comes to the leptin diet. Unfortunately, many people eat lots of carbohydrates during breakfast such as waffles, bagels, cereal and pastries. Despite common misconceptions, this type of breakfast does not give the body an extra boost of energy to get through the day. Eating protein-rich breakfast can boost the metabolism and increase it by as much as 30% for as long as 12 hours, while a carbohydrate heavy breakfast only increases metabolic rate by 4%.

A protein-rich breakfast includes items such as cottage cheese, almond butter, eggs or a smoothie that contains whey protein.

## 2. Eat Three Meals Per Day

It is important to eat three healthy meals a day and not to snack, even though some subscribe to the notion of eating several small meals per day. Allow between 5-6 hours between every meal. This helps clear triglycerides from the blood. When these small blobs of fat build up, they can cause leptin resistance. When you refrain from snacking, the liver jumps into action and naturally clears the triglycerides from the blood. This essential action can only happen if you give yourself the appropriate time between meals for the body to spring into action.

## 3. Keep Your Meals Small

Small meals are one of the big keys to success with the leptin diet. Those on the diet should try to stop eating when they feel only slightly satisfied, not full. Wait around 10-20 minutes, and the " full signal" will eventually catch up. The brain will tell the body that it is full and that it doesn't need any more food. It can take a while at first for the brain and the signal to catch up, but as dieters continue their efforts, the signal will catch up faster.  Keeping meals small is much more important than focusing on the calorie and fat content in a meal.

## 4. Never Eat After Dinner

On the leptin diet, the time that a person eats dinner is just as important as the dinner itself. Those on the diet should never go to bed on a full stomach, they should try to eat dinner at least three hours before you go to bed and should allow approximately 11-12 hours between breakfast and dinner.

## Reduce Your Overall Carbohydrate Consumption

Most of the leptin diet is about eating the right amounts at the right time. However, there is one rule on actual consumption that dieters need to focus on with this diet plan. Leptin dieters do not need to avoid carbohydrates entirely, as the body and the thyroid needs carbohydrates to function properly.

A great rule of thumb is to eat a 50% portion of carbohydrates and 50% protein. The rest of any other meal should be vegetables. Each serving size needs to be around the size of the dieters palm. Carbohydrates can be items such as breads, rice, pasta, potatoes, corn or fruit. When choosing carbohydrates, its best to try to eat healthier carbs such as fruit, whole-grains, brown rice and healthier grains such as quinoa or cous cous.

These five rules are the foundation of the leptin diet. Dieters should start by modifying their current eating schedule around these rules and then focus on adding and removing the right foods.

# What to Eat During the Leptin Diet

For most individuals the biggest part of transitioning to the leptin diet lies in changing what they eat and choosing to eat the right things. Oe of the best ways to know what to eat during the leptin diet is to carefully choose items from these lists of approved natural foods.

Fats
Most people think that fats are a 'no-no' in any healthy diet, but the right fats can be an important part of a leptin weight loss diet. When choosing nuts or nut butters, always choose raw, un-salted, or un-roasted nuts, and always avoid peanuts. Healthy fats come from nuts such as almonds, hazelnuts, pecans, pine nuts and walnuts.

Oils

Oils are an important part of any diet as they can be used for cooking or as seasonings and dressings. Many people use standbys such as vegetable oil, but these oils are not filled with "good" fats. Try almond oil, avocado oil or coconut oil.

Goods High in Omega-3 Fatty Acids
Omega-3 acids are important not only in supplement form, but as part of the diet as well. The best way to get these fatty acids is through fish such as halibut, herring, sardines and tuna. Eggs from algae or flax-fed chickens are also high in Omega-3s.

Protein Powders
Adding protein powder to an all-natural fruit smoothie with almond or coconut milk is a great meal replacement and an important part of a leptin-friendly diet. It can be difficult for dieters to choose the right protein powder with so many options on the market. Good protein powder options include egg, vegetable and whey protein powders.

Tofu
Tofu is a great way to get much-needed protein in the diet, particularly for those who are not meat eaters. Plain, herb and Italian tofus are the best for dieters looking to restore normal leptin function.

## Poultry

Poultry is an important source of protein for a leptin resistant diet, especially since many experts believe that at least 30% of the leptin restoring diet should come from protein. Protein-rich proteins include skinless chicken breast, turkey and chicken sausage and ground chicken or turkey. Poultry should preferably be organic and free range, if possible.

## Other Game

Other game, aside from poultry can be a healthy protein source in the leptin diet. Cornish hens, ostrich, pheasant, buffalo, venison and rabbit are all smart options for this diet.

## Dairy and Dairy Substitutes

Healthy sources of dairy for a leptin resistant diet include goat cheese, non-fat cottage cheese and feta and goat cheese. However, too much dairy can interfere with any healthy diet. Try some substitutes for dairy when it comes to milk consumption. Almond and coconut milk provide even more nutrients than dairy milk without extra bad fats.

These are just some of the "A-list" items that are a big part of a leptin diet. Also, virtually any type of vegetable is also a healthy addition to the diet plan. When it comes to getting good carbohydrates and plenty of extra nutrients as part of a leptin resistant diet, dieters should always turn to vegetables. The right diet can go a long way in helping the body reset and helping these leptin hormones get back to functioning and delivering messages in the way that they are supposed to. These foods are the building blocks of any leptin-friendly diet and can help any person's body get the nutrients they need to keep their system functioning in the best manner possible.

# Sample Meals Leptin Diet

Every person is different, and may have different tastes and preferences. However, when it comes to starting a new leptin diet, a great place to start is to use this sample diet as a reference point. This provides an example of a breakdown of a balanced, healthy diet that can help restore leptin sensitivity and reverse the damages from leptin resistance.

Breakfast:
2-3 scrambled eggs
Sauteed vegetables in coconut oil
Lean chicken sausage or turkey bacon

Lunch:
One piece of salmon or lean chicken breast (6-ounces)
Large avocado
1/2-cup fresh grapes

Dinner:
Grilled grass-fed sirloin with garlic and onions cooked in coconut oil
Spinach salad with fresh chopped red onion, carrots and cucumbers in olive oil or vinaigrette dressing
2 cups fresh steamed green beans

Dieters need to try to refrain from snacking as much as possible and remember to that meals ideally need to be spaced out, with 5-6 hours between each meal. If snacking is a must, these are some healthy snack ideas.

Vegetables dipped in hummus
No-fat cottage cheese
Raw nuts
Green and black olives
Avocado slices or guacamole

Meals such as this can assist in combating leptin weight loss issues as well as leptin sensitivity. Most importantly, these recipes as part of the leptin resistance diet help those who struggle to lose weight finally get the results they have been looking for, far more than calorie cutting alone can.

# Conclusion

For many people today, nothing is as frustrating as their struggles with weight gain, fitness and excess belly fat. The good news for these individuals is that medical researchers may have finally found the root of the problem for the many who try to diet and exercise but simply cannot keep their weight in control. This problem, of course, is leptin resistance.

Leptin resistance is a serious condition and one that may actually be at the cause of many people's issues with obesity. When this "weight loss hormone" is functioning as it should, individuals can expect to see improved fat loss, weight loss and overall health. Understanding the basics of leptin resistance and learning how to treat this hormonal challenge can be the solution that many people search for when it comes to finally controlling their struggles with weight gain.

Over time, with the right diet, exercise and lifestyle changes as part of the leptin diet, many people will start to see a better functioning metabolism, have more natural energy and they will even start to see better results with their weight loss efforts. Since leptin is such an important hormone in the body, chances are these individuals will also start to see positive changes in other areas of their health. Leptin impacts everything from fertility to allergies, mood and immunity function. When these essential hormones are acting in the way they should, any individual can enjoy the benefits of living the healthy, balanced life they were intended to live.

# URGENT PLEA!

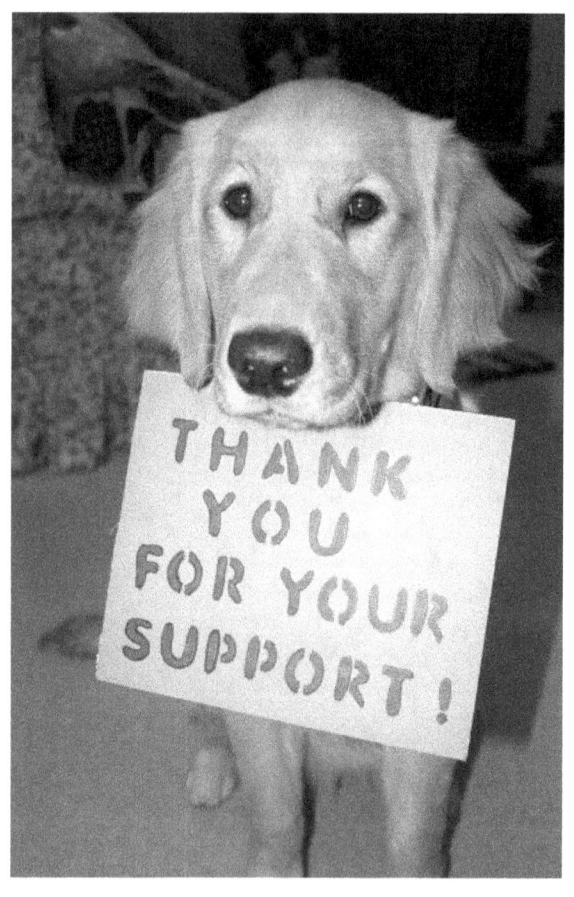

Th an k you for downloading my book!

I really appreciate all of your feedback, and I really like hearing what you have to say. I need your input to make the next version better. Please leave me a helpful REVIEW by turning this page to the very last. Thanks so much!! ~Hanna Krem

## STOP: BEFORE YOU GO
As a Thank You for reading my book,
Claim Your FREE Bonus By
Clicking Below

# SUPER FRUITS and VEGGIES

## 20 Superfoods That Will Transform Your Health

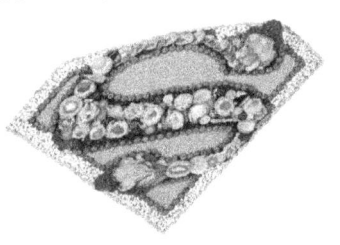

## Hanna M. Krem

Just to say thank you for downloading my book, I would like to give you my 20 Super Fruits And Veggies Report 100% FREE!

Try my other book below, packed with delicious and healthy recipes:

DOWNLOAD NOW

(Or go to http://www.strengthrecipe.com/free)

Seafood Recipes: Ultimate Seafood Soups Under 200 Calories

Paleo Diet: Delicious Paleolithic Recipes For Ultimate Health And Weight Loss

Vegetarian Soup Recipes: Discover Vegetarian Soups Under 200 Calories